Glossary of Terms for
CLINICAL LABORATORY TECHNOLOGY

Glossary of Terms for
CLINICAL LABORATORY TECHNOLOGY

(English-French / French-English)

BRIAN F. HEAD

Copyright © 2018 by Brian F. Head.

Library of Congress Control Number: 2018901920
ISBN: Hardcover   978-1-5434-8479-3
　　　　Softcover   978-1-5434-8478-6
　　　　eBook   978-1-5434-8477-9

All rights reserved. No part of this book may be reproduced or transmitted in any form or by any means, electronic or mechanical, including photocopying, recording, or by any information storage and retrieval system, without permission in writing from the copyright owner.

Any people depicted in stock imagery provided by Getty Images are models, and such images are being used for illustrative purposes only.
Certain stock imagery © Getty Images.

Print information available on the last page.

Rev. date: 02/18/2018

To order additional copies of this book, contact:
Xlibris
1-888-795-4274
www.Xlibris.com
Orders@Xlibris.com

PREFACE

The goal of the initial version of this glossary was utility for a particular purpose: to serve as an aid for Peace Corps volunteers working as laboratory technicians in Morocco. The lexical selection was based on a specific and limited corpus: instructions for a series of laboratory tests prepared by the Ecole des Techniciens de Laboratoire Chimie-Biologique (School for Laboratory Technicians in Biological Chemistry) of the Institut National d'Hygiène (National Health Institute) of Morocco.

The list of lexical items is more detailed than that which is normally found in French-English glossaries of a general technological nature. On the other hand, the list is quite limited, for it was considered feasible, practical, and useful to include only a carefully selected set from among many terms used in clinical laboratory technology. In the selection of items for this list, two criteria were primary: the frequency of occurrence within the corpus used and, in the case of French terms, ease of recognition. The French-English section lists only the most useful terms that are noncognate with English terms along with those which, though cognate, might not be readily recognized. The English-French section lists all technical terms believed to be most useful for Peace Corps volunteers performing the experiments in question in a French-speaking laboratory environment in Morocco, regardless of the degree of cognation. Among the more useful, lengthier lexicons that provide a far greater number of technical terms in this area, but which do not include as detailed a selection of items in the specific fields covered by the present glossary, are *A French-English Dictionary for Chemists* by Austin M. Patterson (2nd ed., New York, 1963), and *French-English Science Dictionary* by Louis DeVries (3rd ed., New York, 1962). This material was prepared in conjunction with the Peace Corps Training Project (Public Health-Morocco) held at the University of Texas during the period August-December, 1964, for which Ernest F. Haden, Rae S. Moore, and the author served as language coordinators. Acknowledgments are due to Nicole T. Head and Sally M. Manning, who, under the direction of the author, translated the original technical material from French into English and compiled a preliminary word list. Much guidance and assistance in the selection of technical terms to be included in this glossary was provided by Curtis Eklund, director of Technical Studies for the project. Arlette Beeckmans, who served as the principal instructor in the phase of training designed for coordination of language and technical studies, further revised and edited the manuscript. The typing was done by Donata Francescato.

The first version of this glossary was not published but instead reproduced by mimeographing. For the present publication, the glossary has been revised, amended, and updated as considered appropriate. The author is responsible for the organization of this glossary and the selection and accuracy of its entries.

Brian F. Head

ENGLISH - FRENCH

A

abnormal	anormal
abscissa	abcisse
absolute	absolu
accuracy, exactness	exactitude
acetic acid	acide acétique
acetone	acetone
acid	acide
acid dye	colorant acide
add	ajouter
adjustment	réglage
agranulocytosis	agranulocytose
air bubbles	bulles d'air
air-tight	hermétique (à l'abri de l'air)
albumin	albumine
alkalimeter	alcalime`tre
alkaline	alcaline
alkalinity	alcalinité
alum	alun
ammonia	ammoniaque

ammonium hydroxide	hydroxyde d'ammonium
ammonium oxalate	oxalate d'ammonium
ammonium thiocyanate	sulfocyanure d'ammonium
analytical balance	balance de precision
anemia	anémie
anhydrous	anhydre
anhydrous sodium carbonate	carbonate de sodium anhydre
anisocytosis	anisocytose
anticoagulant	anticoagulant
aqueous	aqueux
average	moyenne
azur II	azur II
azur II eosin	azur II éosine

B

bacillus	bacille
bacteria	bactéries
balance, scale	balance
ball of the finger	pulpe du doigt

barium chloride	chlorure de baryum
basic	basique
basic dye	colorant basique
basophil	basophile
bead	bille
beaker	bécher
bile	biliaire
bile pigments	pigments biliaires
biological	biologique
biological chemistry (biochemistry)	chimie biologique (biochimie)
biuret reaction	biuret, réaction de ...
bladder cells	cellules du bassinet
blood	sang
blood diluting pipette	pipette à dilution
blood-sugar	glycémie
blue	bleu
blue litmus paper	papier bleu de tournesol
boiling point	ébullition or point d'ebullition
bone marrow	moelle osseuse

brick red	rouge brique
brown red	rouge brun
bubble	bulle
buffer	tampon
buffer solution	eau distillée neutre
bulb	ampoule
Bunsen burner	bec Bunsen
burette	burette

C

calibrated, gauged	jaugé, calibré
capillary pipette	pipette à capillaire
capillary tube	tube capillaire
capsule	capsule
carbolic acid	acide phénique
cells	globule
centrifugation	centrifugation
centrifuge	centrifugeuse
cerebrospinal	céphalo-rachidien
chamber	chambre cellule

check, control	controler
chloride	chlorure
chromatin	chromatine
circuit	secteur
citric acid	acide citrique
clamp	pince
clarified	déféqué
clear	limpide
closed	bouché
clot	caillot
coagulate, coagulated	coaguler, coagulé
coccus	coccus
color	couleur
colored	coloré
colorimeter	colorimètre
colorimetric	colorimétrique
colorless	incolore
compound	composé
condensation	condensation

constitution, composition	complexion
container	récipient
conversion	conversion
converted	transformé
copper sulfate	sulfate de cuivre
cotton	coton
count	numération
to count	énumérar ou compter
counterstain	recolorer
counting chamber	chambre de numération
cover glass, cover slip	lamelle
crenated	crenelé
crystallized	cristallisé
crystallized neutral ammonium sulfate	sulfate neutre d'ammonium cristallisé
culture medium	agent de culture
cuvette	cuvette
cyanmethemoglobin	cyanméthémoglobine
cylinder	tambour

cytoplasm	cytoplasme

D

dark	foncé
dark amber	ambré foncé
decarbonated soda	soude décarbonatée
degree	degré
demand (to), require	exiger
demonstration	démonstration
density	densité
diagnosis	diagnostic
diameter	diamètre
differential	différentiel
dilution bottle	flacon à dilution
dilution (diluting) fluid	liquide de dilution
dilution pipette	pipette à dilution
to discard	rejeter
disease	maladie
dispersion	dispersion
dissolution	dissolution

dissolve	dissoudre
distilled water	eau distillée
distorted image	image parasite
drawing up, to draw up	aspiration, aspirer
drepanocytosis	drépanocyte
drop	goutte
dropping bottle	flacon compte-goutte
to dry	sécher

E

egg white	blanc d'oeuf
electrophotometer	electrophotomètre
element	élément
elliptical	elliptique
enclosed	enfermé
eosin	éosine
eosinophil	éosinophile
eosinophilia	éosinophilie
epithelial casts	cylindres epithéliaux
equivalent	équivalant (équivaloir)

erlenmeyer	erlenmeyer
Erlenmeyer flask	fiole d'Erlenmeyer
erythrocyte	erythrocyte
erythrocyte casts	cylindres hématiques
ethanol, ethyl alcohol	ethanol
ethyl	ethyle
evaluation	évaluation
excess	excès
experiments	procédés

F

factor	facteur
falsify (to), falsifier	fausser
fasting	jeûne
fatty casts	cylindres grasseux
Fehling solution	liqueur de Fehling
fermentation tube	tube à fermentation
ferric	de fer
ferric perchloride	perchlorure de fer
ferricyanide	ferricyanure

filament	filament
filamentous	filamenteux
fill	remplir
filter (glass)	filtre écran
filter paper	papier filtre
filtrate	filtrat
flask, bottle	fiole, flacon
flat	plat
flow	couler
fluid	liquide
formol, formalin	formol
fresh	frais, fraiche
fuchsin	fuchsine
full	plein, pleine
fungus, mold	champignon
funnel	entonnoir
funnel-rack	porte entonnoir

G

gaiac-pyridine	gaiac-pyridine

galvanometer	galvanomètee
gasometric	gazométrique
gentian violet	violet de gentiane
Giremsa	giemsa
glacial	glacial
glitter cells	cellules de sternheimer
glucide, carbohydrate	glucide
glucose	glucose
glycerol	glycérol
glycosuria	glucosurie, glycosurie
graduated	gradué
graduated cylinder	éprouvette
granular casts	cylindres granuleux
granule	granule
greenish brown	brun verdâtre
grid, ruling	grille
grouping	groupement
guaiacum resin	résine de Gaiac
guiding mark	trait repère

H

hydrogen peroxide
hypochromic

hématimètre	hemacytometer
hématocrite	hematocrit
hématologie	hematology
hémoglobine	hemoglobin
héparine	heparine
hétérogène	heterogeneous
homogène	homogeneous
cylindres hyalins	hyaline cylinders
acide chlorhydrique	hydrochloric acid
eau oxygénée	perhydrol
hygroscopique	hygroscopic
hypochromique	hypochromic

I

illuminated	éclairé
impurity	impureté
incoagulable	incoagulable

infection	infection
inflammable	inflammable
insufficient	insuffisant
in use, in practice	pour l'usage, de l'usage
invert	invertir
investigation	examination
iodide	iodure
iron	fer
irregular	irrégulier
irregularly shaped	de forme irrégulière
isotonic	isotonique

J

Jolly bodies	corps de Jolly

L

lavender	lavande
layer, coat	couche
lead	plomb
lens	lentille

leukocytosis	leucocytose
leukopenia	leucopénie
light intensity	intensité de la lumière
light yellow	jaune clair
lilac	lilas
line, mark	trait
liquid	liquide
litmus	tournesol
litmus paper	papier de tournesol
lyse (to)	lyser

M

magnification	grossissement
manipulation, procedures, handling	manipulation
material, equipment	matériel
May-Grunwald stain	may-grunwald dosage
measurements, determination	mesure
medicinal	officinal
mercuric iodide	iodure mercurique

mercurous	mercureux
mercury	mercure
methemoglobin	méthémoglobine
methyl alcohol	alcool méthylique
methylene blue	bleu de méthylène
microburette	microburette
micrococcus	micrococcus
microcytosis	microcytose
mix	mélanger
mixture	mélange
modification	modification
mononucleated	mononucléaire
mononucleosis	mononucléose
morphological	morphologique
morphology	morphologie
mortar	mortier
mouth (relating to the ...), buccal	buccal
mouthpiece	embouchure
mucous	mucus

multiply (to)	multiplier, compter
myelogram	myélogramme

N

needle	aiguille
nephelometer	néphélométre
nephelometric	néphélométrique
neutral	neutre
neutral lead acetate	acétate neutre de plomb
neutrophil	neutrophile
nitrate	nitrate
nitric acid	acide nitrique
nitro-mercury	nitromercurique
non-hemorragic	non-hémorrangique
normochromic	normochromique
normocytosis	normocytose
nucleolus	nucléole
nucleus	noyau
nutrient agar	gélose
nutrient broth	bouillon de culture

O

objective	objectif
oil immersion	huile d'immersion
opaque	opaque
optical density	densité optique
orange	orange
ordinate	ordonnée
ovalocytosis	ovalocyte
oxalate	oxalate
oxide	oxyde

P

parasite	parasite
pathogenic	pathogène
percentage	pourcentage
perhydrol	perhydrol
peri-nuclear, poly-nuclear	péri-nucléaire
periphery	périphérie
permanganate	permanganate

pernicious	pernicieux
Petri plate (dish)	plaque de Petri
phenol	phénol
phenolphthalein	phénolphtaléine
photometer	photomètee
photometric	photométrique
pigment	pigment
pink	rose
pipette	pipette
plate of glass	plaque de verre
platelet	plaquette
poikilocytosis	poikilocytose
poison	poison
polychromatophilia	polychromatophilie
polycythemia	polyglobulie
polynucleated	polynucléaire
porcelain plate	plaque de porcelaine
potassium cyanide	cyanure de potassium
potassium ferricyanide	ferrocyanure de potassium
potassium iodate	iodate de potassium

potassium iodide	iodure de potassium
potassium oxalate potassium	oxalate de potassium
permangate	permanganate de potassium
powder	poudre
precipitate	precipitation
precision balance or analytical balance	balance de précision
prick	piquer
pulverize (to)	pulvériser
pure	pur
purple	violet, pourpre
pyramidon	pyramidon
pyridine	pyridine
precipitate	précipité

Q

quantity	quantité

R

rate	taux

reaction	réaction
reagent	réactif
reagent bottle	flacon à réactifs
research	recherche
recording, record, entry	enregistrement
red blood cell count	numération des globules rouges
red blood cell	globule rouge, hématie
red blood cells	globules rouges hématies
red litmus paper	papier rouge de tournesol
red mercuric oxide	oxyde rouge de mercure
reduced	réduit (réduire)
refrigerator	frigorifère
reject, discard	rejeter
renal cells	cellules rein
epitheliales du reserve	reserve
residual	résiduel
resin	resine
restore (to)	rétablir
reticulocyte	réticulocytaire

rinse	rincer
Rochelle salt	sel de Seignette
rubber	caoutchouc
rubber stopper	bouchon de caoutchouc
rubber tubing	tube en caoutchouc

S

safranin	safranine
salt	sel
sample, specimen	échantillon
screwcap tube	tube à vis
sediment	sédiment
sedimentation	sédimentation
segmentation	segmentation
self-agglutination	auto agglutination
settling, sedimentation	sédimentation
shake (to)	agiter
shape	forme
shutter	volet
sickle red blood cell	hématie falciforme

silver	argent
skin	peau
slide	lame
smear	graisser
sodium bicarbonate	bicarbonate de sodium
sodium chloride	chlorure de sodium
sodium fluoride	fluorure de sodium
sodium hydroxide	lessive de soude
sodium hypobromite	hypobromite de sodium
sodium iodide	iodure de sodium
sodium nitroprusside	nitroprussiate de sodium
sodium sulfate	sulfate de sodium
sodium thiosulfite	hyposulfite de sodium
soiled, dirty	souillé, sale
solvent	solvant
solution	solution
solution bottle	flacon à solution
sources of error	causes d'erreurs
spatula	spatule
spermatozoa	spermatozoides

spherocytosis	sphérocytose
spirillum	spirille
spread	étaler
square	carré
stability	stabilité
stain (to)	colorer
staining bottle	flacon à colorant
standard curve	courbe étalon
staphylococcus	staphylocoque
stemmed glass, test tube	verre à pied
stirring rod	agitateur
stopcock	robinet
stoppered, closed	bouché
streptococcus	streptocoque
subject	sujet
sublimated	sublimé
sulfuric acid	acide sulfurique
supplementary	supplémentaire
swollen	gonflé

T

tap water (stream of ...)	jet du robinet
target cell	cellule cible
tartrate	tartrate
technique	technique
test tube	éprouvette
thin	mince
thiocyanate	sulfocyanure
thiosulfite	hyposulfite
thrombocytopenia	thrombocytopénie
thumb	pouce
tinted	teinté
tip	pointe
title	titre
tourniquet	garrot
transformer	transformateur
translucent	translucide
treatment	traitement
trench, moat, trough	rigole

trichloroacetic acid	acide trichloroacétique
triphosphates	phosphates triples
trough	cuve, rigole
tube	tube
turbid	troublé

U

uncorrected	incorrigé
urates	urates
urea	urée
ureometer	uréomètre
urethral cells	cellules des voies urinaires
urinary albumin	albumine urinaire
urinary glucose	glucose urinaire
urine	urine
use, utilization	utilisation

V

vaseline	vaseline
venipuncture	punction des veines

venous, vein	veineux, veine
vial	fiole
virulence	virulence
volumetric flask	fiole jaugée or ballon jaugé

W

washed	lavé
washed flowers of sulfur	fleurs de soufre lavées
washing bottle	pissette
watch glass	verre de montre
waxy casts	cylindres cireux
weighing, weight (to weigh)	pesée, poids (peser)
well-cleaned	bien propre
white blood cell	globule blanc (leucocyte)
wipe (to)	essuyer
wipe off	essuyer
withdrawal (of blood)	prelévement

Y

yeasts	levures
yellow	jaune
jaune ambré	jellow amber

FRENCH — ENGLISH

A

acétate neutre de plomb	neutral lead acetate
acide acétique	acetic acid
agent de culture	culture medium culture agent
agitateur	stirring rod
agiter	to shake, stir
aiguille	needle
jeun	fasting
ajouter	to add
alcool méthylique	methyl alcohol
ambré foncé	dark amber
ammoniaque	ammonia
ampoule	bulb
anémie	anemia
anneaux de Cabot	Cabot rings
anormal	abnormal
anticoagulant	anticoagulant
aqueux	aqueous
argent	silver

aspiration	drawing up
aspirer	to draw up
auto-agglutination	self-agglutination

B

bactér,ies	bacteria
balance de précision	analytical balance
bec Bunsen	Bunsen burner
bécher	beaker
biliaire	bile
bille	bead
blanc d'oeuf	egg white
bleu	blue
bouché	stoppered, closed
bouchon de caoutchouc	rubber stopper
bouillon de culture	nutrient broth
brun verdatre	greenish brown
buccal	relating to the mouth
bulle	bubble
bulles d'air	air bubbles

burette	burette

C

caillot	clot
caoutchouc	rubber
carré	square
causes d'erreurs	sources of errors
cellule, chambre	chamber
cellule cible	target cell
cellules du bassinet	bladder cells
cellules épithéliales du rein	renal cells
cellules de sternmheimer	glitter cells
cellules des voies urinaires	urethral cells
centrifugation	centrifugation
céphalo rachidien	cerebrospinal
chambre de numération	counting chamber
champignon	fungus, mold
chimie biologique	biological chemistry biochemistry
chlorhydrique (acide ...)	hydrochloric acid

chlorure	chloride
coaguler	coagulate,
coagulé	coagulated
colorant acide	acid dye
colorant basique	basic dye
coloré	colored
colorer	to stain
colorimétre	colorimeter
colorimétrique	colorimetric
complexion	constitution, composition
composé	compound
compter	to count
controler	to check, control
corps de Jolly	Jolly bodies
couche	coat, layer
couler	to flow
couleur	color
courbe étalon	standard curve
crénelé	crenated
cristallisé	crystallized

cristaux de leucine	tyrosine crystals
cuve	trough, tank
cuvette	cuvette (basin, dish, cup)
cyanure de potassium	potassium cyanide
cylindres cireux	waxy casts
cylindres épithéliaux	epithelial casts
cylindres graisseux	fatty casts
cylindres granuleux	granular casts
cylindres hématiques	erythrocyte casts
cylindres hyalins	hyaline casts

D

déféqué	clarified
démonstration	demonstration
dissoudre	to dissolve
dosage	measurement, determination, proportion

E

eau distillée	distilled water
eau oxygénée	hydrogen peroxide

ébullition	boiling
échantillon	specimen, sample
éclairé	illuminated, lighted
électrophotomètre	photoelectrometer
embouchure	mouthpiece
enfermé	enclosed
enregistrement	recording, registration
entonnoir	funnel
énumérer	to count
éprouvette	graduated cylinder
essuyer	to wipe, to wipe dry
exactitude	exactness, accuracy
exiger	to require, to demand

F

fausser	to falsify
fer	iron
ferricyanure	ferricyanide
filtre écran	glass filter, vial
fiole	fiole

flacon	flask bottle
fiole jaugée	volumetric flask
flacon à dilution	dilution bottle
flacon à réactifs	reagent bottle
flacon à solution	solution bottle
flacon compte-gouttes	dropping bottle
fleurs de soufre lavées	washed flowers of sulfur
foncé	dark
formol	formalin, formol
fraiche, frais	fresh

G

gélose	nutrient agar
glacial	glacial
globules	cells
globule blanc leucocyte	white blood cell
globule rouge, hématie	red blood cell
glucose	glucose
glycémie	blood-sugar
gonflé	swollen

goutte	drop
gradué	graduated
graisser	smear
grille	ruling, grid
grossissement	magnification

H

hématie falciforme	sickle red blood cell
hématies	red blood cells
hématimétre	hemacytometer
hématologie	hematology
hémoglobine	hemoglobin
hermétique (à l'abri de l'air)	air tight
hémorragique	hemorraged
hétérogène	heterogeneous
homogène	homogeneous
huile d'immersion	immersion oil
hyposulfite	thiosulfate

I

image parasite	distorted image
incolore	colorless
insuffisant	insufficient
iode	iodine
iodure	iodide

J

jaugé, calibré	calibrated, gauged
jaune	yellow
jaune ambré	yellow amber
jaune clair	light yellow
jet du robinet	jet of tap water, stream

L

lame	slide
lamelle	cover glass, cover slip
lavande	lavender
lavé	washed
lentille	lens

lessive de soude	sodium hydroxide
leucocytes	white blood cells
levures	yeasts
lilas	lilac
limpide	clear
liqueur de Fehling	Fehling solution
liquide	fluid
liquide de dilution	dilution fluid

M

magma	sediment, mixture
maladie	disease
manipulation	procedure, manipulation, handling
materiel	equipment, material
mélange	mixture
mélanger	to mix
mesure	measure, proportion, determination
mince	thin

moelle osseuse	bone marrow
mortier	mortar
moyenne	average
mucus	mucous

N

nitroprussiate de sodium	sodium nitroprusside
noyau	nucleus
numération	count
numération des globules rouges	red blood cell count

O

objectif	objective
officinal	medicinal
ordonnée	ordinate
oxalate	oxalate

P

papier bleu de tournesol	blue litmus paper
papier filtre	filter paper

papier rouge de tournesol	red litmus paper
papier tournesol	litmus paper
paraffine	paraffin
peau	skin
perchlorure de fer	ferric perchloride
pesée	weighing, weight
phénique (acide)	carbolic acid
pigments biliaires	bile pigments
pince	clamp
pipette	pipette
pipette à capillaire	capillary pipette
pipette à dilution	dilution pipette
pipette à dilution, pipette compte-globules	blood diluting pipette
piquer	prick
pissette	washing bottle
plaque de Petri	Petri plate (disil)
plaque de porcelaine	porcelain plate
plaque de verre	plate of glass
plaquette	platelet

plein	full
plomb	lead
pointe	tip
polyglobulie	polycythemia
ponction des veines	venipuncture
pouce	thumb
poudre	powder
pour l'usage	in use, in practice
précipité	precipitate, precipitation
prélèvement	withdrawal (of blood)
propre (bien propre)	well-cleaned
pulpe du doigt	ball of the finger

R

réactif	reagent
recherche	ininvestigation, research, examination
rérecipient	container
recolorer	counterstain
réduit (réduire)	reduced

réglage	adjustment
rejeter	to discard
remplir	to fill
réserve	reserve
rétablir	to restore
rigole	trough, moat
rincé (rincée)	rinsed
rincer	to rinse
robinet	stopcock
rose	pink
rouge	red
rouge brique	brick red
rouge brun	brown red

S

sang	blood
sécher	to dry
secteur	circuit
sédimentation	settling, sedimentation
sel	salt

sel de Seignette	Rochelle salt
solution	solution
soude décarbonatée	decarbonated soda
souillé, sale	dirty, soiled
spatule	spatula
spermatozoides	spermatozoa
sujet	subject
sulfate de cuivre	copper sulfate
sulfate de soude	sodium sulfate
sulfocyanure	thiocyanate

T

tambour	cylinder, drum
tampon	buffer
taux	rate
technique	technique
teinté	tinted
titre	title
tournesol	litmus
trait	line, mark

trait repére	guiding mark
transformé	converted
troublé	turbid
tube capillaire	capillary tube
tube à essai	test tube
tube à fermentation	fermentation tube
tube à vis	screwcap tube
tube en caoutchouc	rubber tubing

U

urée	urea
urine	urine
utilisation	use, utilization

V

veine, veineux	vein, venous
verre à pied	stemmed glass (test tube)
verre de montré	watch glass
violet	purple
volet	shutter

www.ingramcontent.com/pod-product-compliance
Lightning Source LLC
Chambersburg PA
CBHW030907180526
45163CB00004B/1741